The Book on Rheumatoid Arthritis Treatment

Nathan Wei, MD, FACP, FACR
Clinical Director
Arthritis Treatment Center
Frederick, Maryland

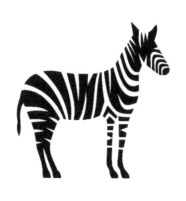

© Copyright Zebra Communications 2010

All rights reserved. No part of this program may be reproduced or utilized in form or by any means, electronic or mechanical including recording, duplicating, or by informational storage or retrieval system without the written permission from the author and publisher.

**Library of Congress
Cataloging-in-Publication Data pending
Wei, Nathan**

Key words: 1. Arthritis Treatment 2. Rheumatoid Arthritis.

This book should not be a substitute for a thorough examination by your physician. The products that are mentioned in this book are recommended. Prior to using any of them, we recommend you seek advice from a qualified specialist. Neither the publisher nor the author may be held liable for any injury, loss, or damage sustained by anyone who relies on the information contained in the book.

Table of Contents

Chapter 1 5
Why Treating Rheumatoid Arthritis Is A Mission For Me

Chapter 2 7
Background Information And Why The Immune System Does What It Does

Chapter 3 14
RA Is A Systemic Disease

Chapter 4 20
Diagnosis: Signs and Symptoms

Chapter 5 26
Diagnostic Procedures

Chapter 6 32
Conventional Treatment

Chapter 7 65
Alternative Treatment

Chapter 8 75
Clinical Research

Chapter 9 77
Brief Notes on Other Things You Should Know

Chapter 10 79
Final Tips

Chapter 11 86
Conclusion

Chapter 1

Why Treating Rheumatoid Arthritis Is A Mission For Me

In the summer of 1968, I traveled to California to look for a summer job. My parents had told me that I ought to visit some relatives while I was there. They said that my great aunt had not been feeling well. But nothing prepared me for what I encountered....

Her hands were crippled and her fingers were tied in knots.

The knuckles were swollen the size of quarters. You would think she was 95, but she was only in her 50s.

She told me it wasn't so bad when she was younger. With the passing years, though, the pain got worse. The arthritis soon ravaged her body.

She said more than once, "If only I had done something about it when I was younger...." But by then it was too late.

I'll never forget the look of agony on her face as she tried to lift her arms. I later learned that it wasn't just arthritis. She'd fractured many bones as a result of osteoporosis from the high doses of steroids used to control her arthritis. Steroids were the only drugs that seemed to work then.

We both broke down in tears as we hugged. She died two months later. My great uncle said the pain just got to her. She couldn't take it anymore and gave up. I also discovered that for a long time my great uncle was the one who did the letter writing. My great aunt told him what to say. He had to write because she couldn't even hold a pen!

Now permit me to fast-forward 15 years to Thanksgiving of 1983. Our whole family was together. My sister, Esther, asked me to look at her feet. They'd been hurting her for several months, so much so that she had given up tap dancing— her favorite hobby. She'd already seen a podiatrist and an orthopedic surgeon, but her feet were still hurting. She took off her shoes, and I took one look. I saw the swelling. I looked at her hands, and…my worst fears were confirmed. My heart sank. She had rheumatoid arthritis!

Despite a rocky, early start, Esther received the proper medical care and –most importantly– aggressive treatment. In 1997 she ran the New York City Marathon in a time of 4 hours and 20 minutes.

Chapter 2

Background Information And Why The Immune System Does What It Does

At one time rheumatoid arthritis was known as "the great crippler."

So... exactly what is rheumatoid arthritis (RA)? Simply defined, it is a chronic, systemic, progressive, inflammatory disease that targets primarily the joints. It involves the small joints of the hands and feet most often, although it can affect virtually any joint in the body. An important feature is RA tends to be symmetric, meaning the joints affected on one side of the body are the same ones affected on the other. The exact cause of RA is still unknown.

Rheumatoid arthritis affects more than 2 million Americans. And worldwide, it affects approximately one percent of the population. Women are affected two to three times as often as men. The peak age of onset is between the ages of 25 and 50.

Although it is not inherited, RA has a genetic component. Family studies show that first-degree relatives have a rate of occurrence that is four times that of the general population. Similarly, if one identical twin has RA, the other twin has almost a 1 in 4 chance of getting the disease. (Mitchell DM. Epidemiology, Rheumatoid Arthritis, Etiology, Diagnosis and Treatment. Edited by PD Utsinger, NJ Zvaifler, GE Ehrlich. Philadelphia. JB Lippincott Co., 1985, pp. 133-150.)

Not that long ago (at least I don't think it was that long ago)—as recently as the 1980s—the anticipated survival for disabled patients with rheumatoid arthritis was 50 percent or less over 5 years...similar to that for patients with three-vessel coronary artery disease or Stage 4 Hodgkin's disease!

And despite the advances made with this disease since that time, delay in treatment still makes disability more likely.

That's because damage in RA takes place quickly—often within the first 6 to 12 months—and this damage can't be reversed. Once the joint is injured or destroyed, that's it. Fortunately, these dismal statistics have changed for the better.

So how does the damage occur?

A typical joint consists of a cavity containing the ends of long bones that have a covering of cartilage. A membrane consisting of cells (synoviocytes) lines the joint cavity. In RA, this synovial lining grows thicker as a result of the multiplication of synovial cells and the infiltration of inflammatory cells.

The development of rheumatoid arthritis is a complex process.

Everything starts with the immune system and what is called the inflammatory response. An acute inflammatory response is a good thing, as it allows us to ward off infection. Sometimes, though, the inflammatory response becomes chronic, and this can cause problems.

The immune system is the body's natural defense mechanism. When any foreign invader (bacteria, for example) enters the body, the immune system goes to work.

Do you remember the game, Pac-man? The little yellow guy that gobbled up things? Well... your body has a special cell called a macrophage that acts just like that. Macrophages are scavengers that attack and gobble up anything that the body recognizes as alien. So these macrophages gobble up foreign particles which are called antigens.

Now... the exact antigen that seems to trigger rheumatoid arthritis is still not known but is suspected to be related to a type of bacteria. Dr. Gerald Weissman at the New York University School of Medicine has developed a hypothesis. He states that an oral bacteria that is a cause of periodontal disease, *Porphyromonas gingivalis*, has an enzyme that creates antigens that lead to joint inflammation.

Also, the macrophage is more than just a scavenger. It's a factory designed to prepare the antigen for digestion. The macrophage first puts that antigen on an assembly line. The first part of the assembly line acts like a Cuisinart, chopping the antigen into small pieces called peptides. The next step on the assembly line is to mix these peptides together with a special part of the macrophage called the human leukocyte antigen (HLA) to make the peptides more "digestible."

This special peptide "appetizer" is called an antigen complex. The antigen complex moves along the assembly line to the "shipping area," which is at the surface of the macrophage. Then the macrophage looks for cells to which it can give this antigen complex. In particular, it looks for a cell called a helper T lymphocyte (T-cell). When the macrophage spots such a cell, it presents the antigen complex to the T-cell—sort of like a house-warming gift! When presented with this "gift" by the macrophage, the T-cell is so grateful that it sheds "tears of gratitude." Better known as cytokines, these tears of gratitude attract more T-cells to the party. These cytokines also alert the neighbors—B lymphocytes (B-cells) and these B-cells are so happy to attend the party that they produce antibodies. These antibodies then help the macrophages gobble up more antigens. In fact, B-cells are no longer viewed as just bystanders in this process. They play an important role in the handling of antigens. B-cells produce destructive enzymes, stimulate other cells to join in, and also interact with T-cells.

This entire process—the recruitment of T and B lymphocytes, the production of cytokines, and the release of antibodies—normally helps a person to fight off infection. But this inflammatory response is in delicate balance.

Unfortunately, the immune system can get its signals crossed when a person who has a vulnerable set of genes comes into contact with a set of antigens that is particularly harmful. The process of inflammation may tip the wrong way and become destructive if uncontrolled.

Remember cytokines…the tears of gratitude? Sometimes, the T-cells pump out these cytokines too fast. Two cytokines are especially harmful at excessive levels: tumor necrosis factor (TNF) and interleukin 1 (IL-1). When overproduced, these two cytokines cause extensive tissue damage. The immune system then begins to gobble up the body's own cells instead of foreign particles. This process is called autoimmunity.

We now know that there are many other cytokines (besides TNF and IL-1) and many other cellular mechanisms involved in the complex process of inflammation. An example of other cytokines that seem to play a fairly significant role are interleukin 6 (IL-6) and interleukin 17 (IL-17). There are many other cytokines that appear to be involved but it is still not clear to what extent.

To summarize what happens in RA…

The contact between a genetically susceptible individual and an environmental trigger—called an antigen—sets everything in motion. We still don't know what the environmental trigger is, but some investigators have long suspected that it is an infectious agent. (Harris ED Jr. Mechanisms of disease: Rheumatoid arthritis pathophysiology and implications for therapy. NEJM 322: 1277-1299, 1990).

The macrophages gobble up and process the antigen; then they recruit lymphocytes to "their party." This recruitment process leads to the excessive production of enzymes called cytokines. While there are both "good" as well as "bad" cytokines, the ones that are produced in excess appear to be destructive. Either these cytokines cause damage by themselves, or they recruit other destructive cells. The result is severe inflammation and a "chewing away" of cartilage, bone, tendons, and ligaments.

Chapter 3
RA Is A Systemic Disease...

Because RA is a systemic disease, it can involve other organ systems, such as the eyes, nerves, heart, lungs, blood, and skin, and contribute to the development of other conditions, such as cancer.

Musculoskeletal complications are the most obvious ones that occur in RA. Inadequate treatment allows progressive joint damage to occur. Ligaments and tendons adjacent to joints can be damaged as well. An example would be the extensor tendons leading to the fourth and fifth fingers. These tendons permit a patient to extend their fingers. Long-standing disease in the wrist can make the end of the ulna (arm bone) jagged and sharp. This saws away at the tendons and they rupture. This complication requires immediate consultation with a hand surgeon.

Patients with RA can develop Sjögren's syndrome, a condition that damages and destroys the glands that make tears and saliva. Complaints of dry eyes and dry mouth are tip-offs to this condition. Ophthalmology consultation is mandatory in order to avoid permanent damage to the eyes.

Rheumatoid arthritis may affect the eyes by causing two conditions: scleritis and episcleritis. Although pain, redness, and irritation are the most common symptoms, these conditions can lead to blindness.

Ironically, treatment can also affect the eyes.

For example, the steroid eye drops that are often given to patients with rheumatoid eye involvement can mask an infection in the eye. Also, long-term steroid therapy can lead to cataracts.

Although RA rarely affects the brain itself, it does affect the cervical spine. And when it does, it can cause huge problems. The relationship between the first two neck vertebrae can become unstable, resulting in pressure on the spinal cord. Unexpected trauma, such as that caused by an auto accident, or manipulation, such as the extension of the neck for the insertion of a breathing tube when a patient must have general anesthesia, can be fatal. Any time that a patient with RA complains of neck pain, it is necessary to obtain x-rays to look for this type of instability. The treatment is a combination of anti-inflammatory medications, analgesics, stabilization of the neck with a soft neck collar, and immediate neurosurgical evaluation.

Another neurologic condition commonly associated with RA is carpal tunnel syndrome. This condition develops when inflammation of the tissues of the wrist exerts pressure on the median nerve leading into the hand. Symptoms of numbness, tingling, and pain in the hand usually involve the thumb and the first two fingers (carpal tunnel syndrome). If not corrected, the pressure on the median nerve can lead to muscle atrophy in the hand. Similar problems can affect the ulnar nerve at the wrist or elbow; patients with this condition complain of numbness, tingling, and pain involving the fourth and fifth fingers, and they have difficulty spreading their fingers apart (ulnar nerve compression).

In other neurologic effects of RA, pinching of a branch of the radial nerve at the elbow can make it impossible to straighten out the fingers. At the back of the knee, inflamed tissue can compress nerves leading into the ankle and foot, and it can pinch nerves at the ankle (tarsal tunnel syndrome). The treatment for these situations is splinting (braces or pads), steroid injections (sometimes using what is termed hydro-dissection technique with ultrasound guidance), physical therapy, and sometimes surgery.

Heart involvement with RA is not as common as it once was… probably because of earlier detection and more aggressive therapy. Inflammation can occur in the heart muscle itself (myocarditis), in the sac that surrounds the heart (pericarditis), in the valves within the heart (non-infectious endocarditis), and in the aorta leading away from the heart (aortitis).

More ominously, patients with RA have an increased incidence of atherosclerotic disease including heart attack and stroke (M.J. Roman, E. Moeller, A. Davis, S.A. Paget, et al. Preclinical Carotid Atherosclerosis in Patients with Rheumatoid Arthritis. Annals Int Med. 2006;144: 249-256). This increased risk is real, serious, and appears to be directly related to the chronic inflammation associated with inadequately treated disease.

Lung disease in RA comes in several varieties. Fluid on the lungs (technically termed pleural effusion) is the most common. Lung tissue itself can be involved with scarring, cavities (holes), and nodules (spots) forming in the lung, and destruction of lung tissue, termed "fibrosis." When RA affects the lung, it may decrease lung function and can become a life-threatening problem. Consultation with a lung specialist is an excellent idea.

Anemia (low red blood cell count) is also common in patients with RA. The anemia can be caused by a number of factors. First, RA itself can cause anemia. This is called the anemia of chronic disease. The more active the disease is, the worse the anemia. Generally, the anemia improves as the disease becomes better controlled. Another cause of anemia in rheumatoid arthritis is medication related. Patients taking non-steroidal anti-inflammatory drugs (NSAIDS) can develop ulcers in the stomach and small intestine leading to either acute or chronic bleeding from the bowel.

A very unusual condition called Felty's syndrome occurs in some patients with RA. These patients have a large spleen, a low white blood cell count, ulcers of the skin (especially on the legs), and a tendency to develop skin infections.

Kidney involvement due to RA is unusual. More often than not, kidney problems are the result of a medication effect. For example, non-steroidal anti-inflammatory (NSAIDS) drugs can adversely affect kidney function. Drugs such as gold and d-penicillamine which were once used commonly also can affect the kidneys as can cyclosporine, an immunosuppressive drug used by some practitioners.

Rheumatoid arthritis is associated with an increased incidence of cancer. The most common type of cancer in patients with RA is lymphoma. (Baecklund E, Ekbom A, Sparén P, Feltelius N, et al. Disease activity and risk of lymphoma in patients with rheumatoid arthritis: nested case-control study. BMJ 1998; 317:180-181). Any patient with swollen lymph nodes, particularly if they complain of night sweats or weight loss, needs immediate oncology evaluation.

Interestingly, RA has a hormonal connection. A well-known and completely baffling situation occurs in women with RA who become pregnant. Most of these women go into remission. Why? Beats me! And it beats a lot of other people, too. Unfortunately, after delivery, the arthritis flares again. For years, a controversy has raged about the effects of oral contraceptives on RA. Some people argue that they protect women against RA, and other people say the effect isn't so great. Who knows?

Chapter 4
Diagnosis: Signs and Symptoms

So how is the diagnosis made?

Because there are so many arthritic conditions, it is imperative to obtain a thorough history and to conduct a careful physical examination. Criteria developed by the American College of Rheumatology help in the diagnosis. (Arnett FC, Edworthy SM, Bloch DA, et al. The American Rheumatism Association 1987 revised criteria for the classification of rheumatoid arthritis. Arthritis Rheum. 1998; 31: 315-324).

These include:

- Joint swelling
- Joint pain
- Symmetry of joint findings
- Morning stiffness
- Fatigue
- Difficulty with movement

Patients' histories can vary a great deal. In two-thirds of patients, the onset of disease is slow, develops symmetrically, and takes place over weeks to months.

Another 15 to 20 percent have an explosive onset of disease; these patients say that "it came on overnight!"

Some patients are incapacitated by their pain… others have to be coaxed to describe what their discomfort is like.

Rheumatoid arthritis patients often have a very high pain threshold since they are so used to living with pain.

Fatigue and morning stiffness lasting at least one hour almost always accompanies the arthritis. Some patients have weight loss, appetite loss, and low grade fever.

And, usually, the key problem that brought patients to the doctor is that they can no longer carry out their normal daily activities!

The progression of RA is fairly typical. Early on, there is swelling and inflammation of the joints. Cartilage begins to deteriorate. Bone begins to erode. If left untreated or inadequately treated, debilitating pain, inflammation, and swelling lead to permanent loss of joint mobility and function. Serious damage can occur in the first year of disease.

X-ray films show joint destruction (a late finding!) in approximately 70 percent of patients by three years.

On examination, rheumatologists look for joint swelling and tenderness that affect small joints mostly—hands, feet, ankles, and wrists. But we check larger joints as well. What arthritis specialists call the cardinal signs of inflammation are swelling, redness, heat, and pain. Any or all of these signs occur at some point during the course of RA. What you don't want to see in patients is loss of function, because this means that they are not going to be able to take care of themselves. A loss of independence can be devastating!

When RA is wreaking havoc…

Damage to joints and surrounding structures, such as ligaments and tendons, can lead to deformities that can affect the patient's ability to perform activities of daily living (Figure 1). These deformities include:

- Swan-neck deformity – when the row of finger joints farthest from the palm, called the distal interphalangeal joints (DIPs), bend and the next row closer to the palm, called the proximal interphalangeal joints (PIPs) extend.
- Boutonnière deformity – when the DIPs extend and the PIPs bend.

- Ulnar drift – when the third row of joints – the metacarpophalangeal joints (MCPs) begin to turn the fingers out.
- Piano-key deformity – when the ulna bone of the wrist becomes very prominent and moves too much.
- Bent-fork deformity – when the wrist bones collapse and the finger bones are forced upward (looks like there is a step down from the hand to the wrist).
- Hallux valgus – when the big toe turns out. Sometimes the second toe crosses over on top of the big toe.

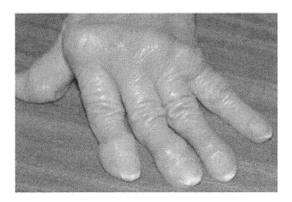

Figure 1 - A rheumatoid hand showing severe deformity.

Even though I've probably said it before, it's worth saying again… it's extremely important to get to the disease before it can do its damage.

The most common complications of RA have to do with joint destruction and deformity, but there are others. For example, patients with positive rheumatoid factors in their blood can develop another problem called rheumatoid nodules (Figure 2).

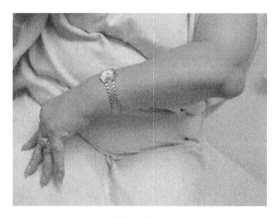

Figure 2

These patients may have lumps of rheumatoid tissue on the hands, feet, elbows, heels (Achilles), top of the feet, or even the back of the skull. Nodules can also develop in the lungs, where they may be confused for cancer! They consist of collections of inflammatory tissue at the site of friction or pressure. Although these nodules usually indicate that the disease has been active for a long period of time, they occasionally appear early in the disease. Any patient who has nodules but whose blood does not contain rheumatoid factor should be suspected of having another disease! Tophi (soft tissue swelling) due to gout can also present with nodules and be a difficult diagnostic problem. Nodules indicate that the RA is a particularly aggressive form of arthritis and requires aggressive treatment.

Another problem is rheumatoid vasculitis. The blood vessels in patients with RA become inflamed. This usually occurs in patients with longstanding or aggressive disease. Men have this condition more often than women do. Most of these patients have rheumatoid factor in their blood. Vasculitis can cause skin ulcers or damage to nerves, and it may reflect internal organ involvement. Skin biopsy is necessary in patients who show signs of this problem. Clearly, this is an indication for aggressive therapy.

Chapter 5
Diagnostic Procedures

Laboratory tests are helpful...

The laboratory is helpful both in excluding other problems and in helping to confirm the diagnosis (Figure 3).

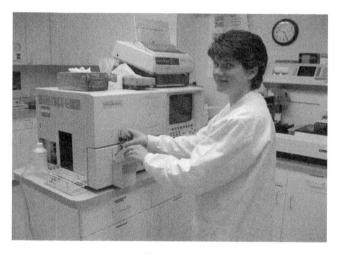

Figure 3

Laboratory testing is critical to making the correct diagnosis. When we see a patient for the first time, we usually order:

- Complete blood cell count (CBC)

- Chemistry panel (This consists of tests that evaluate liver and kidney function)
- Creatine phosphokinase or "CPK" (muscle enzyme test)
- Thyroid function tests
- Erythrocyte sedimentation rate (ESR)
- C-reactive protein (CRP)
- Urinalysis
- Test for rheumatoid factor
- Anti-cyclic citrullinated peptide antibody (anti-CCP)
- Test for antinuclear antibody (ANA)

CPK is helpful since diseases that affect the muscle may also cause aches and pains. These muscle conditions may occur as part of an "overlap" syndrome, meaning the patient has a mixture of conditions. The CPK is useful for telling us if muscle disease is an associated problem.

Thyroid function tests are helpful because thyroid disease is not that uncommon and can aggravate aches and pains.

An abnormal ESR may indicate the presence of inflammation. An elevation of a patient's C-reactive protein (CRP) level has the same significance as an elevated ESR; it suggests the presence of an inflammatory process. Generally, the CRP level goes up and comes down faster than the ESR does.

Anemia often accompanies an elevated ESR, further raising suspicion that the patient has an inflammatory type of arthritis.

Some patients—roughly 80 percent—with RA have rheumatoid factor in the blood. Rheumatoid factor is an antibody directed against another antibody. There are three types of rheumatoid factor: IgM (the most common), IgG, and IgA.

Anti-CCP is a more recently added blood test that is helpful in establishing a diagnosis of rheumatoid arthritis. It is more specific for rheumatoid arthritis than the rheumatoid factor is. If present in a patient at a moderate to high level, it helps confirm the diagnosis of RA. It may also indicate that the patient is at increased risk for damage to the joints.

A positive antinuclear antibody test (ANA), often seen in patients with RA, warrants further evaluation to make sure the patient does not have another condition.

While x-rays are a time honored and useful tool for diagnosis, they do have drawbacks. Erosions (damage to cartilage and bone) may not show up on x-ray for quite some time - months to years. Changes are oftentimes subtle...and open to interpretation. One should not wait around for them to appear!

Newer techniques that include the use of diagnostic ultrasound, magnetic resonance imaging (MRI), and arthroscopic biopsy are helpful. In my opinion, these techniques allow early rapid diagnosis and the institution of aggressive treatment.

In fact, once the diagnosis is suspected, we obtain an MRI of the most affected area—usually a hand, wrist, or foot. We also use gadolinium to aid in the detection of inflammation or erosion/damage to cartilage.

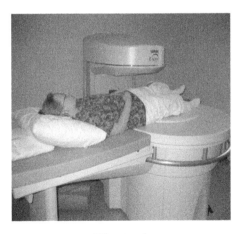

Figure 4

Magnetic resonance imaging is probably the most sensitive and specific means of making the diagnosis (Figure 4).

If magnetic resonance imaging is not available we will use diagnostic ultrasound. Ultrasound is a technique that uses sound waves to image tissue. It is extremely good for detecting early inflammatory changes in the joints. In fact, it may be even better than magnetic resonance imaging in detecting early inflammation. Since it is less costly than MRI it also may have a more practical application in following up on the effectiveness of therapy.

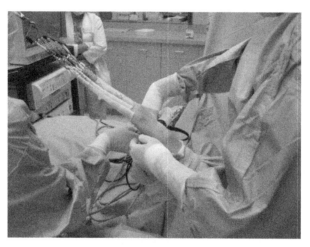

Figure 5 – Arthroscopic biopsy of the wrist in a patient with rheumatoid arthritis.

If we see inflammation of the lining of the joint (synovitis), we then biopsy the joint using arthroscopic guidance to confirm our diagnosis in patients where the disease is suspected but not yet proven (Figure 5).

Arthroscopy with biopsy, particularly in the small joints of the hand and wrist, often reveals unsuspected erosions or erosions that are more severe than that seen on MRI. In our series of more than 300 small joint biopsies, we have never seen an instance in which the arthroscopic picture was more benign than that shown on MRI or x-ray film!

In the future, we hope that tissue sampling will allow us to custom tailor treatment to the individual patient.

How is that possible? We have reached a level of sophistication regarding RA that allows us, in some cases, to tissue type individuals. Patients with certain "biomarkers" may respond to one therapy better than another. In the future, biomarker profiling may be a valuable tool in designing specific therapies.

Chapter 6

Conventional Treatment

Then we get to work...

Prior to 1996, the approach to the management of RA was the traditional treatment pyramid.

Essentially, patients would be started on non-steroidal anti-inflammatory drugs. If symptoms are persistent, steroids would be added. If this doesn't work then the next level up – gold, d-penicillamine, cyclophosphamide and other immune suppressive drugs would be used.

So, treatment would start with the least aggressive, most mild medicines; as the disease progressed over the years, treatment would involve stronger and stronger medicines…usually until the patient had a horrible side effect or was confined to a wheelchair.

The 1996 American College of Rheumatology Guidelines for the Management of Rheumatoid Arthritis shifted our thinking. Although it noted that the ultimate goal of remission is rarely achieved, it outlined several management goals:

- Control disease activity
- Alleviate pain
- Maintain function
- Maximize quality of life
- Slow joint damage

The 1996 approach indicated that the pyramid approach was no longer carved in stone. But this still wasn't good enough, because we began to think...remission is not only possible but often achievable.

So many of us in rheumatology decided to turn the pyramid upside down!

What are some of these treatments?

The first treatment for patients with RA is reassurance and emotional support. The diagnosis can still be a devastating one, and the patient needs reassurance that RA is very treatable. Second, patient education regarding the disease and the medicines being considered are critical. Third, pain and stiffness should be treated.

Anti-inflammatory management

Early on, many patients with RA are placed on non-steroidal anti-inflammatory drugs (NSAIDS). While this is still a part of the early strategy, it is not as prominent as it used to be.

Examples of these NSAIDS include:

- ibuprofen (Advil, Motrin)
- naproxen (Aleve, Naprosyn)
- piroxicam (Feldene)
- sulindac (Clinoril)
- tolmetin sodium (Tolectin)
- indomethicin (Indocin)
- diclofenac (Voltaren)
- etodolac (Lodine)
- nabumetone (Relafen)
- oxazaprocin (Daypro)
- meloxicam (Mobic)

Many of these drugs are no longer in widespread use. These non-steroidal drugs act by blocking a key enzyme called cyclooxygenease (COX). Cyclooxygenase is responsible for converting arachodonic acid, a substance found in cell walls, into prostaglandins.

There are at least two types of COX. The first, known as COX-1, helps produce prostaglandins responsible for certain normal functions in the body, such as protecting the stomach lining and maintaining normal kidney function.

The other, known as COX-2, helps create prostaglandins that cause inflammation. All NSAIDS block both COX-1 and COX-2. Clearly, blocking the enzyme responsible for normal functioning of the stomach lining and kidneys could have harmful effects. And that is what happens.

By blocking cyclooxygenase, NSAIDS help to prevent inflammation; however, they may not be effective enough. And…they may cause substantial side effects due to the inhibition of the prostaglandins responsible for normal body functions.

Among the potential side effects are peptic ulcer disease and gastrointestinal bleeding, fluid retention, liver and kidney dysfunction, platelet dysfunction, bruising, true allergic reactions, weight gain, hypertension, drug interaction, dizziness, drowsiness, and rash.

Newer COX-2–selective anti-inflammatory drugs that block COX-2 only were originally designed to help avoid some of the side effects associated with traditional NSAIDS. The theory was if the "bad"

COX-2 could be blocked while sparing the "good" COX-1, then many potential side effects could be side-stepped. These drugs, when they first arrived, seemed to have fewer gastrointestinal issues; they also had their own set of problems.

Rofecoxib (Vioxx), the first COX-2 drug to get FDA approval, was also the first COX-2 drug to be taken off the market by the FDA. It was found to have an undesirable cardiovascular profile with what appeared to be an increase in heart attack risk.

Valdecoxib (Bextra), another COX-2 drug was also removed from the market by the manufacturer (at the request of the FDA) because of a perceived increase in risk of life-threatening skin problems.

Also, it was noted that patients who were taking aspirin prophylaxis for stroke or heart attack along with their COX-2 drugs had the same risk of gastrointestinal problems as did patients taking NSAIDS alone.

Celecoxib, the only COX-2 drug remaining on the market, has also been under fire but it so far has been able to defend its position. To date, it does not appear to have a cardiovascular profile that is riskier than any other NSAID.

In fact, multiple studies have demonstrated that the cardiovascular risk previously thought to be peculiar to COX-2 drugs appears to be a class effect of NSAIDS in general. (Singh G, Mithal A, Triadafilopoulos G. Both selective COX-2 inhibitors and non-selective NSAIDS increase the risk of acute myocardial infarction in patients with arthritis: Selectivity is with the patient, not the drug class. EULAR 2005; June 8-11, 2005; Vienna, Austria. OP0091.)

Also, rheumatoid arthritis, which is one of the diseases frequently treated with NSAIDS, is itself associated with an increase in cardiovascular risk. Low-dose prednisone (5mg), an anti-inflammatory steroid, is also effective in controlling inflammation. In fact, this route is preferable in many patients because of the relatively good benefit: risk ratio.

Occasionally, in my practice, when a patient presents with very severe disease, we "pulse" them by giving an intravenous dose (1,000mg) of methylprednisolone, a fast acting steroid. This quiets the disease down and buys us time.

Steroids can also be injected into inflamed joints to quiet them down. Use of ultrasound guidance is recommended in order to inject accurately.

Steroids are the prototypical double-edged sword. Although they are extremely effective in suppressing inflammation, they also have a substantial potential side effect profile as the dosage is increased. Side effects include cataracts, weight gain, mood changes, thinning of the skin, thinning hair, facial hair growth in women, poor healing, acne, moon face, suppression of adrenal gland function, aggravation of blood pressure and diabetes, osteoporosis, stretch marks, avascular necrosis (a painful and severe bone disease), muscle weakness, susceptibility to infection…to name a few.

Treatment of rheumatoid arthritis with steroids then is a delicate balance of risks of the disease versus risks of side effects. Used wisely, however, steroids are a tremendous adjunctive therapy.

Controlling inflammation is not enough!

It is not enough to control the inflammation associated with RA. The disease has to be slowed or stopped. That's why we always use disease-modifying anti-rheumatic drugs (DMARDS) in conjunction with anti-inflammatory agents. Disease-modifying anti-rheumatic drugs tend to act more slowly than anti-inflammatory drugs, taking weeks and sometime months to kick in. Examples of some DMARDS are:

Minocycline (Minocin), an antibiotic, is a member of the tetracycline family. It may help in mild disease, but takes one to three months before an effect—if any effect is going to be seen—is noted. (I admit that I'm a closet minocycline user…but only in the very mildest of cases!)

Sulfasalazine (Azulfidine), is a sulfa-based drug that European physicians favor. Usually, patients respond - if they are going to respond - within one to two months. The response is not overwhelming. Potential side effects include a drop in white blood cell count, fever, liver dysfunction, and decline in sperm count. Frankly, I'm not impressed with sulfasalazine. When I go to meetings and talk with my European colleagues, I can't believe we're talking about the same disease. They find it useful as an alternative to methotrexate.

Hydroxychloroquine (Plaquenil), a drug originally used to treat malaria is effective in mild disease. It may take up to 6 months before this drug has an effect. It's generally safe, although it may be harmful to the retina of the eye. It also may cause muscle weakness, sun sensitivity, rash, psychosis, and gastrointestinal upset. I think a drug like hydroxychloroquine is OK if used for very mild disease or if used in combination with methotrexate.

Generally, unless the disease is extremely mild, I don't fool around with drugs like minocycline, sulfasalazine, or hydroxychloroquine.

These drugs are marginally effective, in my opinion, and do not help with more aggressive disease.

Azathioprine (Imuran) is an immunosuppressive drug that is used in some patients with severe disease. In the rare instances when we use it, we combine it with methotrexate. I don't prescribe much azathioprine any more. I believe that other more effective drugs are available. Possible side effects of azathioprine include a drop in blood counts, liver function test abnormalities, gastrointestinal upset, fever, and drug interactions. It, like almost all anti-rheumatic drugs, should not be used in pregnant women!

Cyclosporine (Sandimmune, Neoral) is a disease-modifying drug originally developed for organ transplant patients. In the past, I've combined this drug with methotrexate. Although it is effective for patients with severe disease, I don't prescribe cyclosporine any more. Potential negative side effects of cyclosporine include kidney dysfunction, hypertension, bleeding, tender gums, increase in hair growth, fluid retention, and appetite loss.

Gold salts are another option. These were once the drug of choice and worked remarkably well. When I first started in practice in 1981, I used a lot of gold.

Gold was discovered by serendipity. It was originally designed as a treatment for tuberculosis but found to be effective for rheumatoid arthritis. Gold is given by intramuscular injection. Side effects include bone marrow suppression, rashes, mouth sores, and kidney damage. Prior to administration, it is important to check blood counts and urinalysis. While I don't use gold any more, I do know there are some rheumatologists who do, particularly in Europe.

The disease-modifying anti-rheumatic drug (DMARD) of choice in our clinic is methotrexate. We start methotrexate either orally or intravenously (and sometimes subcutaneously). It is taken once a week on the same day, preferably at the same time of day. We also have our patients take supplemental folic acid, 1 to 2 mg per day, while they're on methotrexate. Folic acid seems to have protective effects against the development of mouth ulcers, a sometimes troublesome side effect of methotrexate.

Methotrexate is an anti-proliferative drug—it blocks rapidly dividing cells from dividing. The theory is that inflammatory cells multiply more quickly than normal cells do and that methotrexate can slow this multiplication effect. Methotrexate also has effects on lymphocytes that prevent these cells from producing more pro-inflammatory substances.

If patients respond well to methotrexate, we monitor them closely and make adjustments in their dosage periodically. All patients who take methotrexate have monthly blood tests consisting of a complete blood cell count and liver function tests. We also check kidney function and order an ESR determination periodically.

Some people have suggested that the interval for monitoring be extended to every six or even every eight weeks. We have had at least four examples in the last two years of patients on long term use of methotrexate who developed a clinically significant laboratory abnormality that would have been undetected had we followed this protocol. Therefore, we continue to recommend laboratory testing every month.

When methotrexate was first used in the 1980s, many rheumatologists (me included) ordered routine liver biopsies. I no longer do so, as it appears that methotrexate, for the most part, is safer for long term usage than we initially thought. The risk of the liver biopsy procedure must be weighed against the potential for methotrexate to cause a problem in the individual patient.

There are potential side effects associated with methotrexate. For example, it may have negative effects on the bone marrow, resulting in low white blood cell and platelet counts; the liver; and the lung. It may also cause nausea, headaches, dizziness, mood changes, rashes, sun sensitivity, hair loss, abdominal cramping, and mouth ulcers. Some patients report that they feel "dragged-out" the day after they take their methotrexate. Hair loss is particularly bothersome for women, and I've had some patients actually discontinue the drug because of this problem.

Shortness of breath or chronic cough should prompt discontinuation of methotrexate to see if it is the cause. If fever and chills accompany the cough, methotrexate should be discontinued immediately. We also have our patients cease taking their methotrexate for a week or two if they have an active respiratory infection or urinary tract infection.

Patients who appear to be at increased risk for side effects associated with methotrexate include those patients who have abnormal kidney function, patients who are folate-deficient, and patients who are taking sulfa drugs. We advise our patients who go on a sulfa antibiotic (such as Bactrim or Septra) for urinary tract infections to hold their methotrexate while they are on the sulfa medication.

Methotrexate is contraindicated in pregnant and nursing women. It is teratogenic and woman should employ strict contraceptive measures. Both men and women who are on methotrexate should discontinue the drug a full three months before trying to conceive children.

Another drug that is used as a DMARD is leflunomide (Arava). This medication has an inhibitory effect on the lymphocytes which induce the RA autoimmune response. It is an oral tablet. Patients may begin with a three day loading dose, then take the drug on a daily basis... or they can just take the oral maintenance dose regularly.

Potential side effects include elevated results on liver function tests, diarrhea, abdominal cramps, aggravation of hypertension, rash, and hair loss. It is also teratogenic (that is, it causes birth defects). I admit that though I used to prescribe leflunomide often, I don't use as much because it doesn't work as well as the biologic therapies. It also occupies a niche.

So what happens if a patient doesn't respond to methotrexate… and how do you measure lack of response?

These are key questions. The presence of response can be quantified using both clinical as well as laboratory criteria. Several methods of measuring clinical response have been written about. One system employs the American College of Rheumatology criteria which assigns a specific score to indicate a patient responding with 20 percent effect (ACR 20), 50 percent effect (ACR 50) and 70 percent effect (ACR 70). There is also an ACR 90 now.

Another scoring system that is used a great deal is the Disease Activity Score or DAS.

Practically speaking, what many practicing rheumatologists use is the age-old "How are you doing"… and "How do you feel" technique which is probably as good as the more formal measurements… and actually has been shown to correlate with the more sophisticated measuring systems, particularly when it is used in conjunction with careful joint exam and laboratory testing.

Now let's talk about what happens if a patient doesn't respond to methotrexate.

If the patient is taking methotrexate and prednisone and does not respond or responds less than we would like to within 4-12 weeks, we then add a biologic response-modifying drug.

The emphasis is on "add." We do not discontinue the methotrexate. And we also continue low-dose prednisone.

Biologic response modifiers act to block cytokines. Remember… cytokines are the chemical signals released by lymphocytes that cause and perpetuate RA. The pivotal cytokine appears to be TNF. Blocking TNF often controls RA. Examples of anti-TNF drugs available are etanercept (Enbrel), adalimumab (Humira) infliximab (Remicade), certolizumab (Cimzia), and golimumab (Simponi).

All of these drugs are effective. Etanercept (Enbrel) was the first FDA approved anti-TNF drug. It was originally derived from the ovaries of Chinese hamsters. It is a protein that binds to TNF alpha. It acts like a sponge to remove most of the TNF alpha molecules from the joints and blood. This prevents TNF alpha from perpetuating inflammation and the pain, tenderness and swelling of joints in patients with different types of arthritis. Etanercept is usually used in combination with methotrexate in patients who do not respond adequately to methotrexate alone. Etanercept comes in two different preparations. The first is a powder that must be reconstituted (mixed) with a diluent. This comes as a 25mg dose. The second is as a premixed syringe containing 50mg of etanercept. Etanercept must be refrigerated. It can be given twice a week subcutaneously— much like insulin. It also can be given once a week in a single 50mg. dose.

The 50mg dose hurts because of the preservative. The makers of Enbrel recently came out with a special pen that may help with the ease of injection. The half-life of etanercept is approximately 92 hours, so patients with severe disease may have a flare-up toward the end of the week. In some cases, it may be necessary to increase the dosage to as much as 75-100mg per week.

The drug has been approved for use in rheumatoid arthritis, psoriatic arthritis, and ankylosing spondylitis.

Since etanercept has entered the market, there have been reports of multiple sclerosis, myelitis, and optic neuritis in patients using the drug. Etanercept is not recommended for persons with pre-existing disease of the central nervous system (brain and/or spinal cord) or for those with multiple sclerosis, myelitis, or optic neuritis. Rare cases of potentially serious low blood counts (pancytopenia) have been reported in patients using etanercept.

It may also, like other drugs in this class, increase susceptibility to respiratory infections as well as lead to reactivation of tuberculosis.

Susceptibility to fungal infections such as histoplasmosis, cocidiomycosis, pneumocystosis, and others is also a problem.

TNF inhibitor drugs should not be administered to patients who have active infections of any sort.

Recently, TNF inhibitors have been shown to cause low blood sugars in patients with diabetes who are taking drugs to lower their blood sugar.

An increased incidence of lymphoma and non-melanoma skin cancers has been observed in patients taking TNF inhibitors.

Adalimumab (Humira) is another anti-TNF drug. It is constructed from a fully human monoclonal antibody. It binds to TNF alpha, preventing it from activating TNF receptors.

It acts like a barrier to the interaction between TNF alpha and receptors for TNF alpha on immune cells. This prevents TNF alpha from perpetuating inflammation and the pain, tenderness and swelling of joints in patients with different types of arthritis. Humira can be used alone or in combination with methotrexate.

It comes in a 40mg prefilled syringe and is administered subcutaneously every two weeks, although some patients may require weekly injections. The only drawback I've heard is that the shot stings (Actually, the 50mg dose of Enbrel does too). Both etanercept and adalimumab come with special kits to help with injection. Teaching by our clinical nurses helps patients feel more confident about injecting themselves. *Humira* also comes as a special injection pen that may make the shots easier.

Serious infections, including tuberculosis, have occurred in patients receiving *Humira*. In some cases, these infections have been fatal. Before starting the drug, and any biologic drug, a patient should be tested for TB. Any medication prescribed for the treatment of TB should start before beginning *Humira* and should be continued until completion.

Since anti-TNF drugs suppress important parts of the immune system, patients receiving these drugs should not be given vaccines containing live viruses.

TNF-blocking agents have been associated with reactivation of hepatitis B.

Some cases have been fatal.

Rare cases of demyelinating syndromes such as multiple sclerosis have been reported as with etanercept.

Anti-TNF drugs should be used with caution in patients with congestive heart failure. This makes for an interesting problem. Since patients with rheumatoid arthritis are at risk for cardiac events such as heart attacks, is it safer to use these drugs or safer not to? This is a question that still needs to be addressed fully.

Combining TNF inhibitors and Kineret (anakinra) is not recommended. The benefit is no greater and the risk of infection is higher.

Pregnancy is a contraindication to TNF inhibitors, as is nursing of infants.

There have been rare cases of severe allergic reactions after taking Humira. The most common side effects associated with Humira are injection site reactions, upper respiratory tract infections, headache, and nausea.

Lymphoma and pancytopenia (low blood counts) have also been rarely reported in patients taking anti-TNF therapy.

While I mentioned that there is an increased incidence of lymphoma observed in patients taking TNF inhibitors, it is not clear whether the occurrence of lymphoma is any higher in patients taking TNF inhibitor drugs than in patients with RA alone. In fact, there is some possible evidence that TNF inhibitors make actually reduce the incidence of lymphoma in RA patients.

Infliximab (Remicade) is a monoclonal chimeric antibody (part human, part mouse) directed against TNF alpha. Infliximab is approved for use alone or combined with methotrexate for treating moderate to severe rheumatoid arthritis. It also is approved for the treatment of active psoriatic arthritis and ankylosing spondylitis.

Infliximab is administered intravenously. The recommended dose for the treatment of rheumatoid arthritis is 3mg/kg as a single dose. The initial dose should be followed by additional 3mg/kg doses two and six weeks after the first dose. The maintenance dose depends on the patient's response. It can be increased to a maximum of 10mg/kg every four weeks. The most common side effects of infliximab are upper respiratory tract infections, urinary tract infections, cough, rash, back pain, nausea, vomiting, abdominal pain, headache, weakness and fever. Infusion reactions, which are sometimes severe, may occur.

Side effects such as fluctuations in blood pressure, chest pain, difficulty breathing, rash, itching, fever and chills may occur during or shortly after administration. These reactions could possibly be due to an allergy to the drug.

They are more common among patients who develop antibodies to infliximab and are less likely to occur in patients who are taking drugs that suppress the immune system, such as methotrexate. Infliximab should be discontinued if serious reactions occur.

Infliximab should not be used in patients with serious infections. Infliximab should be discontinued if a serious infection develops during treatment. Before starting infliximab, as well as with other TNF inhibitors, patients should have tuberculosis skin testing, because of reports of reactivation of tuberculosis in patients taking these drugs.

There have been rare cases of serious liver injury in people taking infliximab.

Screening for hepatitis B is mandatory.

Infliximab should not be used in patients with congestive heart failure or other significant heart disease.

Approximately half of infliximab treated patients in clinical trials developed a positive ANA during the trial compared with approximately one-fifth of placebo-treated patients. Anti-double-stranded DNA antibodies (antibodies found in systemic lupus erythematosus) were newly detected in approximately one-fifth of infliximab treated patients compared with zero percent of placebo-treated patients. Reports of lupus and lupus like syndromes, however, remain uncommon.

Decreased white and red blood cell and decreased platelet counts have been reported with infliximab. Vasculitis (inflammation of arteries) also has been reported.

As mentioned earlier, patients with rheumatoid arthritis, particularly patients with very active disease and/or chronic exposure to immunosuppressive therapies, may be at a higher risk (up to several fold) than the general population for the development of lymphoma. It is not known whether anti-TNF therapy raises or lowers this level of risk.

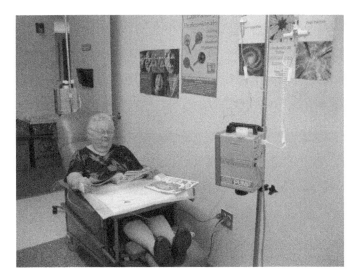

Figure 6

At our center, we have a special infusion room equipped with infusion supplies, a "crash cart," a television, and comfortable chairs (Figure 6).

Cimzia is one of the newer TNF inhibitors. It is formed by covalently joining the TNF inhibiting protein with polyethylene glycol (PEG), a nontoxic, nonimmunogenic polymer approved by the US Food and Drug Administration for use in foods, cosmetics, and pharmaceuticals.

Conjugation with PEG, termed PEGylation, modifies the structure and function of the parent protein, resulting in a compound with improved therapeutic capabilities. (Material from the *Cimzia* website).

This PEGylation process seems to keep the drug inside the joint longer, increase the time inside the circulation, and improve stability of the drug. (Harris JM, Chess RB. Effect of pegylation on pharmaceuticals. *Nat Rev Drug Discov.* 2003;2:214-221).

Cimzia can be administered as a subcutaneous injection either as 200 mg every two weeks or 400mg once a month.

Simponi is the fifth TNF inhibitor. It is a human monoclonal antibody directed against TNF. It comes either in a prefilled syringe or an auto-injector pen. *Simponi* has the advantage of once monthly subcutaneous dosing- 50mg. The only problem is that sometimes there is dosage creep and patients need to take the drug a bit more often than once a month.

Simponi is also FDA approved for treating psoriatic arthritis and ankylosing spondylitis.

The potential toxicities and side effects of *Cimzia* and *Simponi* are similar with this medication as with the other TNF inhibitors.

Some patients respond to one anti-TNF drug; some, to another. Oftentimes, the patient's insurance status dictates the drug used, as these drugs are very expensive. Insurance companies sometimes balk before agreeing to pay for these drugs. For this reason, we always contact the patient's insurers to get authorization before starting therapy.

Anti-TNF drugs slow down the rate at which RA damages joints and bones.

Studies have also indicated biologic response modifiers reduce pain, inflammation, and stiffness, and improve range of motion. An improvement in energy and activities of daily living may also occur.

Is there a difference among the various TNF agents as far as efficacy? Probably not.

And as far as we know, all five agents can be used as first line TNF therapy.

To sum up the potential side effects again... infusion reactions (hives, itching, shortness of breath, chest pains) and reactivation of tuberculosis (more common with infliximab than the other anti-TNFs, it appears), infectious complications, aggravation of congestive heart failure, rashes, injection site reactions, and rare reports of demylelinating illness (similar to multiple sclerosis).

We go through a checklist before starting therapy with biologic response modifiers. We check for the following:

- History of severe congestive heart failure (This is a relative contraindication to therapy with biologic response modifiers.)
- Presence of lymphoma
- Active infectious disease
- Other exclusionary criteria such as hepatitis

Patients with the following medical conditions require extra special monitoring:

- Mild heart failure
- History of multiple sclerosis
- History of cancer

Before starting anti-TNF therapy, we make sure that patients have had all their needed vaccinations and elective surgery.

Because of the potential for reactivation of tuberculosis as a result of anti-TNF therapy, we also have all patients get a tuberculosis skin test.

This is called a PPD skin test. Patients with a positive result on the PPD skin test also get a chest x-ray and/or a computed tomography (CT) scan of the chest. We encourage consultation with a pulmonary disease specialist.

To prevent reactivation of tuberculosis, some experts recommend treatment with isoniazid in patients whose PPD skin test has a positive result.

Controversy exists as to when patients receiving anti-TNF therapy should also receive isoniazid prophylaxis.

If a patient does not respond to one anti-TNF agent or begins to lose their responsiveness to their present agent, we will switch them to another. There is a chance they will respond to the second or even the third.

Case history: A 29-year-old executive secretary came in with a six month history of generalized morning stiffness and the recent development of swelling in the hands and wrists. She also had more fatigue than usual. Physical examination showed some very mild swelling in the hands and wrists with some tenderness. Laboratory tests showed a mildly elevated ESR and a low level of rheumatoid factor. A diagnosis of rheumatoid arthritis was made. An MRI study showed evidence of mild inflammation in one of the wrists. An arthroscopy showed severe synovitis and the presence of erosions. The patient was started immediately on low dose prednisone, methotrexate, and etanercept. She went into complete remission within four weeks.

Another anticytokine drug, anakinra (Kineret), blocks interleukin 1. It seems to be less effective than the anti-TNF drugs and our experience with this medication has not been all that encouraging. Anakinra is self-administered subcutaneously daily. Combining anakinra with anti-TNF drugs does not make it any more effective than anti-TNF drugs alone and may even lead to more side effects! (Genovese MC, Cohen S, Moreland L, Lium D, et al. Combination therapy with etanercept and anakinra in the treatment of patients with rheumatoid arthritis who have been treated unsuccessfully with methotrexate. Arthritis Rheum. 2004; 5 (50): 1412-9). I don't use Kineret because I don't think it's very effective.

For patients who don't respond to any of these drugs, there are other options that we consider. The first is second generation biologic therapies.

These include rituximab (Rituxan), tocilizumab (Actemra), and abatacept (Orencia).

Rituximab (Rituxan) works by targeting B-cells. B-cells manufacture the antibodies which go haywire in autoimmune disease. Numerous studies have demonstrated the pivotal role of B-cells in the pathogenesis of RA.

Rituxan is a sterile, clear, colorless, preservative free liquid concentrate for intravenous (IV) administration. Rituxan is administered intravenously and is given as an intravenous infusion two times during a two week period of time and then not given again for 6 to 12 months. There's still no real consensus as to whether a patient should receive the drug regularly at six months or spaced out at other intervals.

The infusions are relatively slow and there are potential side effects including infusion reactions consisting of a drop in blood pressure, elevated heart rate, shortness of breath, rash, and other symptoms commonly seen with infusion related therapies.

Patients are generally given methylprednisolone and Benadryl before they receive their Rituxan to help prevent infusion reactions. Methotrexate is usually continued while patients are taking *Rituxan*.

Side effects with *Rituxan* are similar to that of other biologic therapies with one major exception. *Rituxan* has been reported to cause progressive multifocal leukoencephalopathy (PML). This is a rare inevitably fatal neurologic disease due to activation of the Jakob Creutzfeldt virus.

Signs of PML include confusion, dizziness, speech difficulty, problems with walking, and visual problems. Patients who have been treated with rituximab and develop new neurological signs or symptoms should be evaluated for PML.

Abatacept (CTLA4–Ig) (*Orencia*) is a novel fusion protein designed to modulate the T-cell co-stimulatory signal. This pathway may be critical in the interaction that occurs between the T-cell and the macrophage. It also appears to decrease certain populations of T-cells that are responsible for continuing inflammation.

Clinical trials have provided preliminary evidence of the efficacy of this compound in the treatment of rheumatoid arthritis.

It is given according to body weight. Patients weighing less than 60kg (about 120 pounds) receive 500mg over 30 to 60 minutes. Patients weighing 60-100 kg get 750mg and patients weighing more than 100kg get 1,000 mgs.

The drug is given as an initial dose, then one at two weeks and then once monthly.

Infusion reactions are unusual although hypersensitivity and anaphylaxis have been reported. Common side effects include nausea, respiratory tract infections, and headache. The usual problems with infections seen with other biologics are also an issue with *Orencia*.

Patients with obstructive lung disease appear to be at higher risk of side effects. Effects of immunizations may be blunted. Combining Orencia with TNF inhibitors is not recommended since there is no benefit and there is an increased risk of side effects.

Methotrexate is usually continued while patients are taking Orencia, although data from at least one study indicated that Orencia can be used as monotherapy (by itself without methotrexate).

A new version of *Orencia* that can be given by subcutaneous injection performed as well as the current intravenous formulation. The injectable biologic was equivalent to the intravenous formulation in a pivotal 1,457-patient trial.

The same equivalence was seen with a fixed, 150mg dose of the subcutaneous formulation, whereas the intravenous form, as mentioned above, has to be adjusted for the patient's body weight.

Tociluzamab (*Actemra*) is a humanized (human protein only) antibody directed against the interleukin 6 receptor. In other words, it is an inhibitor of interleukin-6. Interleukin 6 is a key stimulator of inflammation. *Actemra* has been shown in multiple studies to be more effective than either methotrexate or placebo for the treatment of rheumatoid arthritis.

It is given as an intravenous infusion once a month. The infusion lasts about an hour or two. The initial dose is 4mg/kg. If a patient doesn't respond to this dose, then the dose can be increased to 8mg/kg. Common side effects with Actemra include upper respiratory tract infections, headache, and hypertension. Among the other common side effects are elevation of lipids and liver function test abnormalities.

Other serious side effects of *Actemra* include tears of the stomach and intestines, hepatitis B infection in those already carrying the virus, nervous system problems, and serious allergic reactions.

Actemra appears to be most useful in patients who have failed TNF inhibitors. Like many other biologics it works best when combined with methotrexate, although it can be used as monotherapy (by itself).

There are a number of biologic therapies which are undergoing investigation.

The first is ALD518. Like Actemra, it inhibits the action of interleukin-6. However, it does it by a different mechanism. ALD518 is a humanized antibody directed against IL-6 itself, not the receptor. In clinical trials this drug was found to be superior to methotrexate. Side effects included liver function test abnormalities, increases in cholesterol, and drops in white blood cell count.

Other drugs, called "small molecules" are being evaluated.

The most recent of these drugs are the protein kinase drugs. There are three major compounds being researched. They are JAK inhibitors and a SyK inhibitor.

Using what is called messenger RNA, these drugs create a scrambled message that confuses the immune cells so they can't keep on causing problems.

These medicines were a hot topic at the 2010 American College of Rheumatology meeting. JAK has attracted increasing interest as a drug target in rheumatoid arthritis because it's pivotal to the inflammatory response. It's an enzyme that serves as the traffic director for the release of tumor necrosis factor and other cytokines (protein messengers) that accelerate inflammation in diseases such as rheumatoid arthritis. The weakness of JAK is that it is an enzyme whose effects can be blocked by an oral, small molecule drug. There are three forms of JAK simply known as JAK 1, JAK 2, and JAK 3. Pfizer has a JAK inhibitor called tasocitinib. Earlier reports from the ACR meeting about this compound showed that it was extremely effective as well as possessing an acceptable safety profile. Tasocitinib blocks JAK 1 and JAK 3. Tasocitinib is taken twice a day.

Another JAK inhibitor, called INCB028050, is a product from the *Incyte* company. *Incyte* has partnered with Eli Lilly to manufacture and market this compound. The drug produced ACR20 responses (at least 20 percent reductions in symptom scores) in up to 70 percent of patients after 24 weeks, and ACR70 responses in nearly 30 percent of patients, reported Maria Greenwald, MD, of Desert Medical in Palm Desert, Calif. INCB28050 selectively blocks JAK 1 and JAK 2. INCB28050 is taken once a day.

Side effects of the JAK drugs include elevations in both HDL and LDL cholesterol of up to 25 percent, depending on the dosage. Other side effects that have been seen in the clinical trials with these medicines include an increase in respiratory tract infections, viral infections, including shingles, drops in white blood cell count, increases in platelet count, and slight abnormalities in both kidney and liver function.

The SyK drug has similar effects and side effects although maybe more hypertension than the JAK drugs.

Chapter 7
Alternative Treatment

"Your food shall be your remedy. Let food be your medicine and let medicine be your food..."

These words were uttered by Hippocrates.

With all the emphasis on natural remedies currently, one area of great interest is the use of food based oils to help with different disease processes, particularly arthritis.

Most American diets are high in oils called omega-6 fatty acids (linoleic acid) which eventually are broken down to arachodonic acid, which is a cornerstone of inflammation... obviously, not something that is desirable.

So if that's the bad oil, what are the good ones?

One good oil is omega-3 which helps to reduce inflammation. Another good fatty acid is gamma linoleic acid or GLA.

Fish oil is the source of omega-3 fatty acid that has been studied most carefully. Numerous studies have demonstrated its effectiveness in reducing the risk of cardiovascular events as well as reducing the inflammation that accompanies rheumatoid arthritis (RA). Fish oil is available as both a liquid or as a softgel capsule. The typical daily dose is 3 grams per day of EPA/DHA, the active ingredients in fish oil.

If you would like to get your dose of fish oil naturally, you can eat the following types of fish: salmon, tuna, sardines, herring, and mackerel. Omega-3 is abundant in cold water fish.

Another good oil that contains high amounts of GLA is evening primrose oil. Another good source of GLA is borage seed oil. These preparations have been shown to help with the symptoms of RA. Dosage for RA is 1.8 grams of GLA per day.

Another oil that increases the amounts of EPA is flaxseed oil. Flaxseed oil can be used in salad dressings. Flaxseed flour can be used to make baked products.

When purchasing products it's important to read the labels carefully. The packaging should be in opaque containers. Try to get high potency capsules.

Also, be wary of potential side effects. Fish oil and GLA can thin the blood. This is particularly a problem in patients who are taking non-steroidal anti-inflammatory drugs (NSAIDS), blood thinners like

Coumadin, or other herbal remedies such as ginger which can thin the blood also.

Be patient. It takes at least three months before you will notice a benefit.

Some patients do develop gastrointestinal side effects such as gas or heart burn. Also, burps will have a fishy smell. Fish oil can also be excreted with sweat so that you may smell like the local seafood market.

Do not use these oils as your only therapy for RA. It's important to realize that these oils are complementary (used in addition to) conventional medications.

In addition to the above advice, try lowering the amount of red meat you eat. Red meat is high in ingredients that promote the inflammatory process.

Because omega-3 supplements are available without prescription, they are not covered by insurance.

Other dietary supplements for which there is some evidence of beneficial effect for rheumatoid arthritis are:

Black currant oil (*Ribes officinalis*): Major source of ALA (alpha-linoleic acid) and GLA (gamma-linolenic acid). ALA is an omega-3 fatty acid that, to a limited extent, can be converted in the body into two other important omega-3s — EPA (eicosapentaenoic acid) and DHA (docosahexaenoic acid)

GLA is an omega-6 fatty acid. The body ordinarily is able to produce sufficient GLA from the essential fatty acid linoleic acid (LA), which is found in foods containing oils from corn, sunflower, safflower, soy, peanut and other plants, including flaxseed.

Seed oils from black currant, borage, and evening primrose are among the few that are rich in GLA.

Mediterranean diets, which are associated with a lower risk of coronary artery disease and certain types of cancer, are high in ALA. However, the beneficial effects of EPA and DHA (which include cardiovascular benefits and reduced pain associated with rheumatoid arthritis and menstrual cramps) have not been seen with ALA alone. Black currant oil, which has mixture of both ALA and GLA may, consequently, have anti-inflammatory effects due to its GLA content.

GLA may be useful in diseases that involve inflammation. It may also have some benefit in treating rheumatoid arthritis (especially as purified GLA and when combined with traditional treatments) and Raynaud's phenomenon. Many other potential uses, including some in conjunction with fish oils, have been explored, but evidence is either weak or very preliminary.

Black currant seed oil:

This type of oil has the ability to reduce prostaglandin production. (Wu D, et al. Am J Clin Nutr 1999 Oct; 70(4):536-43). This contains 6-19 percent gamma-linolenic acid (GLA). GLA is an omega-6 fatty acid that has potent anti-inflammatory properties. This lessens joint pain and stiffness as well as swelling. One placebo-controlled trial in 56 patients with rheumatoid arthritis showed that patients taking GLA for six months had significant improvement in joint pain, stiffness, and grip strength (Belch JJ, et al. *Ann Rheum Dis* 1988;47:96-104). GLA was safe. GLA can thin the blood so if you're on a blood thinner, use caution.

Borage oil:

Borage oil comes from the Borage plant. Borage is an annual plant that grows wild in the Mediterranean countries and is cultivated elsewhere. The hollow, bristly, branched and spreading stem grows up to two feet tall. It contains 20-26 percent of the fatty acid GLA. Oils containing the omega-6 fatty acid gamma linolenic acid (GLA)—borage oil (Pullman-Mooar S, et al. *Arthritis Rheum* 1990; 33:1526–1533; Leventhal LJ, et al. *Ann Intern Med* 993;119:867–73; Zurier RB, et al. *Arthritis Rheum* 1996; 39:1808-17)—have been reported to be effective in the treatment for people with RA. The effects are similar to that for black currant oil, i.e., it has anti-inflammatory properties.

Bromelain:

This is an enzyme derived from pineapples and is important for pain free movement of joints. Bromelain is an anti-inflammatory that has been shown to reduce joint swelling but without any side effects. How does it help? Bromelain *(Anas comosus)* inhibits "bad" prostaglandin production and reduces inflammation (*Japanese Journal of Pharmacology*, 1972, vol. 22). Bromelain has long been a mainstay for treating muscle injuries (Blonstein J. *Practitioner* 1960; 203:206), yet now it is believed its anti-inflammatory actions may also ease arthritic pain. The enzymes obtained from the stem of the pineapple *plant (Ananas comosus)* help break down scar tissue, decrease tissue fluid called edema, and block inflammation (Ako H, et al. *Arch Int Pharmacodynamics* 1981; 254:157-67).

Curcumin (*Curcuma longa*):

This is related to the ginger root and has been shown to block prostaglandin production and stimulate the release of cortisol, which together inhibit inflammation. Curcumin is the active constituent of turmeric, the key ingredient found in many curry dishes, which gives curry its distinct color and flavor. Turmeric has been used in Ayurvedic and Chinese medicine for centuries. Clinically, it was found to improve stiffness of joints, morning stiffness, walking time, and joint swelling. It has been shown to help in two studies involving OA and RA. (Ammon HP. *Wien Med Wochenschr* 2002; 152 [15-16]:373-8, Amala Cancer Research Centre, Amala Nagar, Trichur. *Indian J Physiol Pharmacol* 1992 Oct;36 [4]:273-5).

The amount of curcumin usually used is 400mg three times per day (Kulkarni RR, et al. *J Ethnopharmacol* 1991; 33:91-5; Deodhar SD, et al *Ind J Med Res* 1980; 71:632-4).

Evening primrose (*Oenothera biennis*):
This contains GLA. A randomized controlled study showed significant reductions in anti-inflammatory medication needs in patients with RA. (Belch JJF, et al. Ann Rheum Dis. 1988; 47:96-104).

Frankincense:
It's also known as Boswellia serrata. Frankincense has been used as a healing herb. It is found primarily in North Africa. This herb may have anti-inflammatory properties and has been used for treatment of arthritis in Middle Eastern culture for centuries. It's been shown to provide relief in both OA and RA in clinical studies (Chopra A, et al. *ArthritisRheum* 1996;39:S283; Chopra A, et al. *Arthritis Rheum* 1998;41:S198).

Garlic (*Allium sativum*):
A study of patients with RA showed that 87 percent of the garlic treated patients showed a good response. While this was not a

randomized controlled trial, the results are encouraging (Denisov LN, et al. Tereapevticheskii Arkhiv 1999; 71:55-58).

Ginger:
This is another Ayurvedic herb used to treat people with arthritis. A small number of case studies suggest that taking 6 to 50 grams of fresh or powdered ginger per day may reduce the symptoms of RA (Srivastava KC, et al. *Med Hypoth* 1992; 39:342-8.) This root is anti-inflammatory and analgesic. It blocks the production of both leukotrienes as well as prostaglandins.

Green-lipped mussel:
This is a New Zealand shellfish, from which an extract has been shown to be useful in the treatment of rheumatoid arthritis and osteoarthritis. Green-lipped mussel inhibits inflammation in the body.

Although inflammation is normal under certain conditions, consistent or excessive inflammation can result in pain and damage to the body, including the joints. The human body makes several chemical mediators of inflammation. Levels of these chemicals in the body may be higher in people with RA who are experiencing symptoms than in symptom free people with arthritis.

Evidence indicates that controlling the production of inflammatory mediators in the body may help improve conditions such as arthritis, asthma, psoriasis, and inflammatory bowel disease (including ulcerative colitis and Crohn's disease), all of which involve elements of inflammation (Gursel T, et al. *Prostaglandins Leukot Essent Fatty Acids* 1997;56:205-7, Henderson WR Jr. *Ann Intern Med* 1994;121:684-97). In one trial, both freeze dried powder and lipid extract of green-lipped mussel were effective at reducing symptoms in 70 percent of people with OA and 76 percent of people with RA (Gibson SLM, et al. *Comp Ther Med* 1998; 6:122-6). A similar study of people with either OA or RA showed green-lipped mussel reduced pain in 50 percent and 67 percent of the patients, respectively, after three months of supplementation (Gibson RG, et al. *Lancet* 1981; 1:439, Whitehouse MW, et al. *Inflam Pharmacol* 1997;5:237-46).

Thunder god vine:
Chinese herb used for centuries. It may have pain relieving properties. The vine has leaves and flowers that are toxic. Use caution. Lipsky demonstrated this vine may have anti-inflammatory properties. (Lipsky PE, et al. *Semin Arthritis Rheum* 1997; 26:713-723). The fact that the research was done by one of the better known scientists in basic research gives this a lot of credibility.

Turmeric:
This is a yellow spice often used to make curry dishes. The active constituent, curcumin, is a potent anti-inflammatory compound that protects the body against free radicals. A double-blind trial found curcumin to be an effective anti-inflammatory agent in RA patients.

While nutritional supplements and herbs can be valuable adjuncts, they do not take the place of conventional therapies. They used to be used in conjunction with them. That is the reason why alternative therapies are often referred to as "complementary" treatments.

Chapter 8
Clinical Research

The other excellent option for arthritis is participation in clinical trials. The Arthritis Treatment Center has a very active clinical research division with many promising second, third, and fourth-generation biologic response modifiers available.

Patients are offered the option of participation in our research programs. Although some patients are concerned about the possibility of receiving placebo, it must be noted that the placebo response in RA clinical trials can be as high as 30 to 40 percent!

A benefit to the volunteer participating in a clinical trial is that they pay either little or nothing for all study-related expenses.

Almost all of the currently available medicines for rheumatoid arthritis were first evaluated at the Arthritis Treatment Center in clinical trials!

Advantages of participating include:

- Study related medications and procedures at little or no charge to the patient
- First crack at newer medicines
- Skilled and careful evaluation during visits
- An opportunity to help others by volunteering

Chapter 9

Brief Notes on Other Things You Should Know

On occasion, as mentioned in a previous chapter, a patient has a few stubborn joints that remain bothersome and clinically inflamed. Steroid injection often helps. Any joint can be affected in RA, and almost all joints are accessible to injection.

We use diagnostic ultrasound (sound waves) to ensure proper location of our injections (Figure 7, 8).

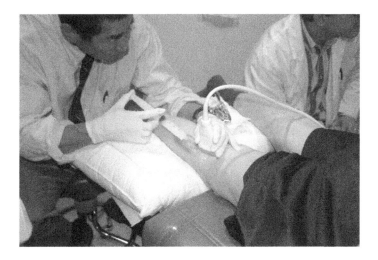

Figure 7 (Ultrasound guided injection)

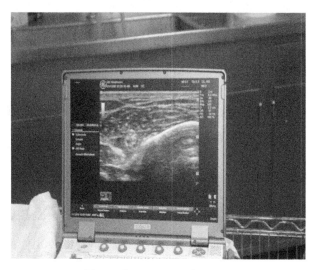

Figure 8 (Ultrasound image)

When a stubborn joint does not respond to steroid injection, we perform an arthroscopic debridement procedure. This offers palliative relief.

Chapter 10
Final Tips

Other therapies that we use and which are pretty simple but very important are...

Patient instruction in proper approaches to the activities of daily living, including such advice as the following:

- Maintain proper posture. Stand straight with your knees slightly bent. Do not slump your shoulders or lock your knees. If you have to stand for a long time, put one of your feet on a stool.

- When sitting, support your body with a lumbar roll. Keep your hips, knees, and ankles at 90 degrees. Use a footrest, if needed. If you work at a desk, keep your seat at the right level. This is a level that permits you to view your monitor at eye level. Use a seat that is a bit higher if you have problems getting into and out of your chair; adjust your seat. Use a book stand to prevent neck strain.

- Use a neck pillow to avoid stressing your neck. Avoid using pillows under your knees, because this will cause knee contractures that will prevent you from straightening out your knees.

- Use multiple pillows to cushion your body, when necessary.

- Use larger, stronger joints to take the load off smaller joints. For example, use a fanny pack or backpack instead of using your arms or hands to carry things.

- Use your palms instead of your fingers to carry things or lift things. Hold items close to your body. Slide objects rather than lift them.

- Change positions as often as possible.

- Do not make any sudden movements or do any lifting if you've been relatively immobile for a time. Ease into it.

- Watch your weight. Excess weight means extra stress on your joints.

- Get organized so that you can do your activities with the least strain and least movement possible.
- Listen to what your body is telling you. If you're hurting, stop.

- Oscillate. Pace yourself so that you do your work and exercise and then rest! This is particularly true if your symptoms are severe. Rest should be adequate, but too much rest can increase stiffness and limit muscle use and activity.

- Use assistive devices, such as splints, to help you with your activities of daily living.

- Use walking aids such as canes and walkers to reduce pain and stress on joints and improve mobility.

- In the kitchen, use electric devices rather than manual ones. An example would be a jar opener or an electric can opener.

- Use rubber jar openers.

- If you're often using gripping implements, look for implements that have a larger handle.

- Try using disposable items to decrease clean-up.

- Ask for assistance in opening jars, or use rubber grips or even pliers.
- Store things within easy reach.
- Use long-handled appliances if they help you avoid bending over.
- Always use convenience items. These are items that help you perform your activities of daily living more efficiently and with less pain.
- Sit on a stool in the bath or shower.
- Use joint-friendly levers instead of faucet handles that require you to turn with your fingers.
- Use grab bars.
- Use a free-standing mirror so you don't have to lean over.
- Wear loose-fitting clothes.
- Use long-handled shoehorns.

- Use a zipper pull.

- Consider Velcro fasteners for your clothes.

- Use light-weight tools with built-up handles.

- Use elastic shoelaces.

- Physical therapy can help with joint flexibility and pain. Physical therapy modalities that are particularly effective include ultrasound, electrical stimulation, and sometimes massage.

- Occupational therapy can help with functional activities at work and at home.

- Exercise therapy, consisting of strengthening, stretching, range-of-motion, and flexibility training, along with balance and coordination may also be helpful. For patients who have RA involvement of weight-bearing joints, water exercise and swimming are good choices. Use of a stationary cycle or elliptical trainer and walking may be acceptable for patients who don't have weight-bearing joint dysfunction.

- Dietary counseling can help maintain ideal weight, plus a careful evaluation for food allergies that may play a role in aggravating the patient's condition.

  Although their limited mobility may make it difficult for some patients to cook and shop for food, it is important for them to maintain a balanced diet. An ideal diet is one that is one that is low in fat, high in fiber and complex carbohydrates. Examples will include: beans, fruits, vegetables, and whole grains. Dietary fish oil may reduce inflammation. Calcium-rich foods are also helpful in maintaining bone health and strength.

- Techniques to reduce stress (e.g., cognitive behavioral therapy, meditation, biofeedback, yoga, Tai Chi).

- Supplemental treatments, such as massage, warm baths containing therapeutic Epsom salts, electric blankets, heating pads, and topical ointments may help.

- On rare occasions, we use mild narcotics such as propoxyphene or acetaminophen with codeine.

- Patients who have had RA for several years may require joint replacement. Fortunately, surgical remedies have advanced to the point where these procedures are effective in improving lifestyle and patient function.

In summary, it is highly unusual not to find an effective therapy or therapies for patients with RA.

Chapter 11
Conclusion

We rheumatologists also may take a page from the oncologists. They use biologic agents, and they use combinations of therapies—each therapy is designed to block a different step in the disease process.

As our knowledge of the mechanisms of disease improves, our ability to target specific problems will improve as well. Because there is a genetic component to RA, there may be a time when we will be able to tissue-type all patients and know immediately which drug will work best for that individual. At that time, we will be close to our Holy Grail—a cure!

New treatment protocols designed to send RA into remission, work effectively, but… only if the patient is diagnosed and treated early and aggressively! Rheumatoid arthritis does not have to be feared today. But it must be respected as a wily and dangerous enemy. Successful treatment hinges on expert management by rheumatologists who have the courage, knowledge, training, and facilities to treat this condition with the attention it deserves.

For more information about arthritis, contact:

The Arthritis Treatment Center
71 Thomas Johnson Drive
Frederick, MD 21702
(301) 694-5800
www.arthritistreatmentcenter.com

If you want to know more about Rheumatoid Arthritis go to http://rheumatoidarthritistreatmentandrelief.com/RAbookoffer/ password: arthritis" for the Second Opinion Arthritis Treatment Kit (SOATK).

The definitive collection of information on both conventional and alternative therapies for arthritis. Here's some of what you'll discover…

- Discover five myths about arthritis that could cause you unnecessary vicious pain…
- Is it arthritis… is it bursitis… or tendonitis… the diagnosis is critical and here's why…
- Finger joint lumps and bumps… what are they?
- Foods to shun so you shrug off arthritis pain.
- The new super treatments that reverse rheumatoid arthritis.
- Best osteoarthritis remedy of all? This ultra-healing natural method stimulates self-repair!
- Common pain reliever, promoted as harmless, can trash your liver. Take it with alcohol… and die!
- Hocus-pocus magnet therapy? Discover the truth inside these pages.

Each chapter deals with a separate type of arthritis condition… and provides you with the information that will give you back your life.

Get 50 percent off the regular price of the SOATK.

Copy the following link on to your internet browser to take advantage of these incredible savings today!

http://rheumatoidarthritistreatmentandrelief.com/RAbookoffer/

password: arthritis

Made in the USA
Las Vegas, NV
17 March 2022